# WHAT IS BIPOLAR DISORDER

# What Is Bipolar Disorder

Everything About Bipolar Disorder From Understanding Bipolar Disorder Symptoms To Treatment

**Bill Bryanson**

Copyright © 2013 by Bill Bryanson

ISBN-13: 978-1481241397

ISBN-10: 1481241397


All rights reserved. This book or any portion thereof may not be reproduced or used in any manner whatsoever without the express written permission of the publisher except for the use of brief quotations for the purpose of book reviews or articles, without the prior written permission of the publisher.

Book published by Well Being Valley. Well Being Valley is a publishing house which focuses on books relating to physical and mental well-being.

# TABLE OF CONTENT

**THE BIPOLAR CONDITION** .................................................................. 1

**CHAPTER ONE: WHAT IS BIPOLAR** ................................................ 3

    Understanding The Medical Side of Bipolar ................................. 5
    Do You Suffer From Bipolar? ............................................................ 8
    What Causes Bipolar? ..................................................................... 12
    Risk Of Bipolar? ................................................................................ 15
    Seeing A Doctor ............................................................................... 16
    Whom Assistance Should I Look For? ......................................... 18

**CHAPTER TWO: DECIDING IF YOU SHOULD NEED HELP** .... 25

    The Stress Goes Farther ................................................................. 29

**CHAPTER THREE: UNDERSTANDING YOUR DOCTOR'S BIPOLAR TREATMENT** ......................................................................... 33

    Using Medications .......................................................................... 35
    Psychotherapy Treatment .............................................................. 42
    Using Electroconvulsive Therapy ................................................. 46
    What's Right For You? ..................................................................... 49

**CHAPTER FOUR: THE REASON WHY PEOPLE STRUGGLE WITH BIPOLAR TREATMENT** ........................................................... 51

    When The Patient Doesn't Take The Medication ....................... 53
    Other Reasons ................................................................................. 61

**CHAPTER FIVE: HOW TO COPE WITH BIPOLAR DISORDER** .. 63

CHANGE YOUR SLEEPING PATTERNS .................................................................. 65

MEDICATIONS .................................................................................................... 67

STAY ACTIVE ..................................................................................................... 70

STOP USING DRUGS OR ALCOHOL ...................................................................... 71

GET SUPPORT .................................................................................................... 74

LOOK TO REDUCE STRESS .................................................................................. 78

BE ON THE LOOKOUT FOR SIGNS ....................................................................... 82

KEEP IN CONSTANT CONTACT WITH YOUR DOCTOR ............................................ 87

**CHAPTER SIX: HOW SUPPORT GROUPS CAN HELP YOU ......... 91**

DO YOU HAVE A SUPPORT GROUP? .................................................................... 93

GETTING EXTERNAL SUPPORT ............................................................................ 95

**CHAPTER SEVEN: MONITORING SYMPTOMS USING A MOOD CHART ........................................................................................................ 99**

**FINAL NOTES ON BIPOLAR ......................................................................... 103**

**RESOURCES .................................................................................................... 105**

# The Bipolar Condition

Bipolar is a common condition which causes a lot of problems for those who have it. Anyone who suffers from it would tell you that it creates a lot of problems in their lives. If you suffer from this condition, there are high chances that your family would suffer with you. If you suffer from this condition or have a family member who suffers from this condition, there is still hope.

Just to be clear, there is no cure for bipolar yet. However, you can take many measures to live a long and fulfilling life. It doesn't have to change your world apart and isn't too difficult as well. As like all people in day to day life, we all face ups and downs. This is life. We may be all joyful one day and the next day we have problems and feel down.

In this book, you would learn how to deal with many situations which people with bipolar face. You will ultimately learn to cope with bipolar and that constant feeling of ups and downs. Through a deeper understanding of your condition and better help in dealing with your day to day tasks, you will be able to significantly improve your quality of life of you and your loved ones.

# Chapter One: What Is Bipolar

Every bipolar patient that I know has this one goal to live a normal life. They want to get through the day without having any emotional problems. They want to get through the day without people wondering what is wrong with them and to simply enjoy the small joys in life like your son's football game or dinner with their family. However, many patients struggle to do so.

Before you could fully learn to cope with this situation, you need to understand your condition fully. You need to understand why some things happen, so you would use those coping mechanisms to work for you. We would talk deeper about coping mechanisms in the future chapters.

Before I give you any false hopes, I would like to remind you that there is no 100 percent sure way of stopping these things from happening to you. What this book is predominantly focused is to assist you in improving your outlook. To get to this point, I would start giving you some invaluable information about your condition so you would better understand what is truly happening to you.

Regardless of whether you are a family member who want to help or a sufferer, this information would be invaluable so that you would learn whatever is needed to deliver the help that you could give to them.

# Understanding The Medical Side of Bipolar

Bipolar is the medical condition where there are extremes in moods and life experiences. It is without a doubt that bipolar is a serious health condition that creates an extremely difficult situation for those who have it. It is a mental illness and it requires necessary treatment.

Those who have done slight research on bipolar may have heard of the term Manic Depression or that the person suffers from manic depression. However, what scientists have learned is that manic style behavior is only an extreme of this condition. The other part is of depression. Both these conditions are vitally serious to your well-being and must be treated instantly.

While medical researchers haven't got a cause for bipolar, they are working very hard to find for a good reason as to why something like this could happen to a human being. From scientists to doctors, many people in the medical field are working tirelessly to ensure that a cure could be found.

However, until that happens, you would need to learn how to cope with bipolar. For most patients, bipolar starts during their teens. Some groups of medical researchers believe that this condition is mainly triggered by puberty. Other people would develop this condition until they are in their adult years or could even last a life time too.

For a majority of individuals, bipolar is a condition which doesn't happen all the time. It is rather a condition with happens now and then. You don't go in and out of moods or other experiences within a few minutes and you don't do this all of the time. As an example, some people will have bipolar bouts that last for several weeks while others would have them for a few months at a time. It is very rarely that someone with bipolar have flared up symptoms all the time.

Bipolar is a condition that would only worsen if you don't get help. It is without a doubt that depression by itself is a killer. However, not getting help is really a foolish thing to do. Be aware that there are medications, treatments and therapies that could help you reduce symptoms and help you cope with your condition better.

# Do You Suffer From Bipolar?

Firstly, you would need to determine if you actually have this condition. Learning the signs and symptoms would assist you in deciding whether to seek out medical attention. If any of your symptoms are severe or considering hurting yourself, you would need to seek immediate medical attention. Bipolar people would go through alternating patterns of highs and lows of their emotions.

The highs are called episodes of mania while the lows are called episodes of depression. The intensity of the highs and lows would vary from person to person from one episode to another. For some people, symptoms would be quite mild but for others would be quite severe. During the manic phase, there would be some symptoms that could be observed.

- Optimism which couldn't be explained. You would feel an indescribable feeling of euphoria or an inflated self-esteem.
- You would have poor judgment and you may only realize this after you have made the wrong decision.
- You would have incredible fast speech. Your mind would be filled with thoughts that you couldn't understand. You would feel agitated and feel the need to move around constantly.
- Spike in aggressiveness in your behavior.
- Reckless decision making.
- Sleeping problems.

Those people that suffer from the mania of bipolar would transition from it into the depressive side. The symptoms of depressive bipolar include:

- You may feel very tired and feeling uninterested about getting things done. You would lose interest in things that you do daily.
- Feeling sad and guilty for no reason. Feeling hopelessness is also a very common feeling. The feeling may be unfounded and persistent.
- You may feel very irritable and lose your temper for no reason at all.
- You may have trouble sleeping although you are extremely tired.
- You may be hungry constantly and lose weight because you don't eat well.
- You may feel pain that there is no real reason for.
- You may feel suicidal.

It is without a doubt that the worst symptom is the feeling of suicide. If you have such thoughts, you would need immediate attention. Even if you have any of these symptoms, seeking treatment has to be done immediately.

# What Causes Bipolar?

Every bipolar patient that I know wants to know why it happened to them. As doctors, this would be probably the one thing that is most difficult to explain to them.

*Why is this happening to me?*

*Why would I have to go through all these?*

*What can't I just live a normal life?*

Unfortunately, no one could answer that. Medical researchers have been spending many years trying to understand the reasons for bipolar but to no avail. The only good news is that some researchers are able to find some ideas as to why bipolar happens.

Many people in the medicine profession believe that bipolar happens because of a combination of factors. This includes genetics, biological and the environment that one is in. Doctors believe that such conditions wouldn't only cause the onset of bipolar but would also control when you experience the symptoms as well as the frequency of it.

The problem with bipolar is often associated with the brain. There are chemical messengers within your brain that go between nerve cells and the brain itself. The main task of these is to relay information. They are called neurotransmitters. Those who have bipolar have a different chemical messengers and simply communicate in a different way to the brain triggering the symptoms.

It is often believed that those who suffer from bipolar have a certain genetic code which puts them in that situation. While this disposition doesn't actually trigger the condition to happen, per say, those that have this coding have a better chance of developing it at some point in their lives.

That difference between neurotransmitters is believed to be because of the abnormal aspect of the genes. The genes that control the neurotransmitters in your brain simply developed abnormally, causing the bipolar situation. Additionally, doctors believe that is would be necessary that some environmental effects would have to happen to trigger this problem. From drug abuse to dealing with stressful events, all these become reason for the trigger.

# Risk Of Bipolar?

The best way to gauge your risk of bipolar would be your family history. If your family has a strong history of bipolar or other depressive conditions, you may be at high risk for it as well.

In fact, a medical research that was done said that up to 90 percent of those suffering from bipolar have evidence of such conditions in their family. Again, the genes are a very important factor here.

While there is no research that has found the exact gene that causes this, researchers are still spending a tremendous amount of time in finding the gene that causes it.

# Seeing A Doctor

You would have probably realize how important it is to seek medical attention for bipolar. Many people who have bipolar symptoms don't realize it until they have a problem.

Many people will realize that something in their life is probably not right but wouldn't even know that there is such a condition. They aren't aware just how troublesome these mood swings are for their family members. You would perhaps have no idea the trauma that your family and friends are placed if you are under this disorder.

Therefore, it often takes someone else to help you realize that you have such a condition. It is only them that would be able to get you to see a doctor so you could be properly diagnosed for your own sake. Those who care about their loved ones should assist their loved ones seek medical attention if they realize how much they are suffering. Professional help can be incredibly helpful to those who are suffering.

If someone suffers from bipolar but doesn't seek out the help he/she needs, he/she will only continue stressing himself/herself. Not only that, physical problems would also increase and they may even hurt themselves because of the emotional turmoil.

# Whom Assistance Should I Look For?

Upon realizing the need for professional help, you should first contact your family doctor. He/she could help you determine if there are any other medical conditions which cause your condition. From there, you should decide to see a psychiatrist.

Don't worry about the shame that is often associated with seeking diagnosis for medical conditions. In my experience, many patients are ashamed to seek help when they are faced with a mental condition. Understand that you are there because you have a problem and there are many people who have the same problems. The process of seeking help is a very simple one to do.

Take a loved one with you so you would feel more comfortable. Explain to them about the issues that you face. Commonly, the doctor would first ask you about the symptoms that you are experiencing. He/she would ask you to describe the symptoms; from the depressive to the mania ones.

During the initial meeting with your doctor, talk about your day to day lifestyle, the problems that you have and your overall health condition. From there, the doctor would have a better idea on your medical problems and other mental health problems. Other conditions such as emotional disorders, hyperactivity disorder or personality disorders could have similar symptoms to bipolar conditions.

Your doctor may also ask you to go for certain tests to determine if they may be other factors which cause your condition. He/she would want to find out if you have other physical causes for your bipolar disorder.

This may include talking about substance abuse. You will need to be honest to your doctor about things like this. If you use alcohol or other forms of drugs; you would need to tell your doctor about these things. Remember, your doctor is the one that you have to be completely honest to if you want to improve your physical condition. These forms of drugs can have the ability to alter the mood and creates bigger fluctuations of moods.

Another common reason for your mood swings could be because of health problems like thyroid disorders. For such conditions, a blood test would be required. Blood test would determine how well your thyroid is working. Many people that have mood swings actually have a thyroid which is under-active. The good news from here is that if this is the problem, then there are medications that could help treat thyroid problems.

However, there is still more to talk about with your doctor. You would want to tell him about the medications that you are taking as they could also cause a number of mood swings. You should also be aware that if you use medications for your depression or anxiety, it could very easily lead to extreme mood swings.

Most doctors would also ask you more about your diet. The food that you partake will also lead to the number of nutrients that you get. Research had clarified that those people who take diets which lack B12 vitamins in particular could experience vast mood swings.

If you have any of such conditions, you doctor may decide that you are truly suffering from bipolar disorder. He will have a better idea if you truly suffer from such conditions if you are able to tell him your entire lifestyle.

Therefore, honestly communicate with your doctor. Don't be afraid to talk about everything in your life. Even your sex life, if it's needed. They are all very good indications of the life you are living. It will help him make a better decision to treat your current conditions.

It may surprise you that your doctor may even be pretty experienced in dealing with bipolar disorder. This is mainly because there are many people who are diagnosed with this condition. It isn't some condition which is rare and only few people have it. Once you have been actually been diagnosed with bipolar, only then can the doctor work on an appropriate treatment for you.

# Chapter Two: Deciding If You Should Need Help

Unlike a cold that would go away, bipolar is a mental illness. You don't expect bipolar to go away after some time. There is no healing mechanism that would automatically heal your bipolar over time. Without the attention of a professional doctor, your bipolar condition would only get worse over time.

The uniqueness of this condition is that you would have no way of knowing if your condition would worsen quickly or at all. However, research shows that those that do not seek help for their condition would create complications that would not only make it tough for themselves but their family members as well.

You also need to know that other conditions could make your bipolar even worse. If you are trying to deal with anxiety, you would have a hard time doing so because of bipolar. In many conditions, this can be very life threatening.

If you are a user of alcohol, this could also be a serious problem. If you can't keep yourself of alcohol, you would find your life in danger. Not only would alcohol cause additional problems for you, but it would also make you think irrationally and put yourself in a very dangerous situation. For this reason, seeking help is a must.

In many circumstances, the length of time between depressive symptoms and mania could be very short. You could easily move from one symptom to the next quickly, leading to extreme confusion and feeling like you have a big medical problems. This rapid cycle will cause great amount of grief for someone who isn't sure of their situation.

You could get into a terrible state of depression and mania at the same time. When this happens, the end result is that your mind and emotions are completely wrapped in each other. When such things happen, the end result is that your mind is completely wrapped with unexplainable emotions. You feel easily agitated and annoyed. You would feel unable to sleep or eat. You just can't seem to get your thoughts organized.

The worse to come from this would be suicidal thoughts. This is a common situation because the emotions that you have is so tough that you have no way of explaining it. You wouldn't have the ability to think rationally at all and can make some terrible decisions.

Psychosis is also another major problem among bipolar patients. When someone has a tremendous situation of both mania and depression, it leads to psychosis. Psychosis is a very serious mental illness which your personality is completely disorganized. You are impaired by what is real and false. You become hallucinated and delusional. This is a symptom that is very hard to be diagnosed, even by professionals.

# The Stress Goes Farther

Perhaps the most difficult part of being someone with bipolar is the stress that it would place on your relationships. People with bipolar would face a tremendous problem with holding onto relationships. They may easily move from one person to the other quickly because of the mood swings that they deal with.

Additionally, those who suffer from bipolar often make mistakes when dealing with others. Because of their condition, they are often confused about their own true emotions in relation to others.

From here on, many people with bipolar make unwise choices when it comes to everyday decisions from spending their money. They may end up in bad financial problems. I have even see people needing to file bankruptcy to having to burden their family with these financial problems.

In dealing with their topsy turvy emotions, they may sometimes end up in a shopping spree.

However, none of the problems are as bad compared to the way they treat themselves. I have seen situations where people completely isolate themselves from everyone in order to cope with their condition. This is especially so during the depressive phases.

Without this protection from their loved ones, they allow their suicidal thoughts take control. Because of this isolation, it becomes important for loved ones to provide them with the right care to make them feel safe.

It can be clearly understood that the complications of bipolar could be quite severe. Because of the ignorance of this condition, many simply don't realize at all that they have it. It can easily escalate and put other people in danger in the things they do daily.

Bipolar patients are also advised against driving a car. If he/she suffers a mania or depressive mood change, the person would easily lose control of the car and be a problem on the road. They may put other road users in danger.

If you think about it, bipolar is something that could affect your life in all areas. Because we are all emotional human beings and bipolar being an emotional problem, people with bipolar could bring problems to just about anywhere. Therefore always seek appropriate treatment.

Getting help isn't just something that improves your own outlook of life but would also reduce the risks of other people around you as well.

# Chapter Three: Understanding Your Doctor's Bipolar Treatment

After thoroughly discussing with the doctor about what is affecting you, you would need to take some time to understand the treatment that your doctors would recommend to you. This is important if you are looking to cope with your bipolar illness.

Broadly speaking, there are two main forms of treatment. They are medication and psychotherapy. This combination has been known to help many people improve their lives even though they still suffer from bipolar.

I would want to repeat this again. There is no cure for bipolar. There are only treatments that would improve the condition. All treatments are merely coping mechanism to improve your quality of life and to ensure that you are safe.

I would highly recommend this combination as well. In the next few pages, I would explain both of these. From then on, we would talk about what other things that you could do beyond your doctor's care would help you accelerate your improvement.

# Using Medications

There are various medications that your doctor could prescribe to help you. The main purpose of medications to assist you in regulating your mood swings.

Among the most popular forms of medications for mood control include Lithium in brands such as Lithobid and Eskalith. They work as a tool to stabilize your mood and are actually the main tools to work against manic episodes. They would become your first line of defense when you face mood swings.

Additionally, you can also use anti-seizure medications to provide the help that's needed. These medications also do the same purpose of stabilizing your moods. Medications of such nature include valproic acid with brands such as Depakene and Iamotrigine.

The purpose of such medication is to provide the role of mood regulators. A less commonly used anti-seizure medication is Topiramate which is sold as Topamax.

However, you need more help to control the mood swings that are brought about by bipolar disorder. You would probably face multiple episodes of depression and doctors would find it extremely important to handle these symptoms carefully. They could be treated in many ways and you would need to discuss them with your doctor.

The doctor may decide to give you antidepressants. They are especially ideal for treating depression specifically and could often work with bipolar patients.

He may decide to give you antidepressants. Antidepressants are ideal for treating depression specifically and therefore often work with bipolar patients. These medications include:

- Paraxetine (Paxil)
- Buprpion (Wellbutrin)
- Fluoxetine (Proza and Sarafem)
- Sertraline (Zoloft)

Your doctor may also provide you with antipsychotic medications if he feels that you need them. This includes two types:

- Risperidone (Risperdal)
- Olanzapine (Zyprexa)

There are certain medications that are created to treat both depressive and mania symptoms that you face with bipolar disorder.

However, there are often major concerns when using medications in treating bipolar.

There are constant debates about the health risks that would arise when you take them.

For example, the American Diabetes Association has done tremendous research on these commonly used medications and found some serious risks when using them. They have found that the use of antipsychotic medications greatly enhanced the development of diabetes. You would also easily gain weight if you don't have the right exercise and diet. You may also increase your blood pressure because of your increase in weight.

However, it doesn't mean that you couldn't take the medications that your doctor asks you to take. As a matter of fact, you must take them if your doctor asks you to take them. The reasons I am bringing up such issue is just to highlight the importance of understanding the risks of partaking these medications. Needless to say, you should always follow the recommendations of your doctor with regards to your medication, diet and exercise.

Certain medications like Risperdal, Zyprexa and Seroquel are only used in severe bipolar conditions. Even then, when you are using such medication, you have to use them only with the doctor's monitoring. This helps minimize the risks of complications at bay even when you take the medications regularly.

You should also be clear that every medication you take would have different side effects and reactions. Certain people wouldn't react towards certain medications while some people would end up having severe side effects.

When you first start taking these medications, it is absolutely essential for you to consider how each medication could possibly affect you. You can know this by doing your own research or asking your doctor. If you find the side effects absolutely overwhelming or provide too bad a side effect, quickly contact your doctor for advice.

You would also need to realize that medication often require some time before you can see any results. Some medications would take weeks of taking them before you notice any benefits.

If you take the medications but don't see any substantial improvement, talk to your doctor and see what he says. You may decide to try another form of medication or increase the dosage. It takes some time before your doctor would be able to get the perfect dose for you. Be extremely patient during this period and work with your doctor closely so you can gain the benefits from the medication.

# Psychotherapy Treatment

To be clear, psychotherapy isn't a scary thing. It is something that could be done easily if you understand what it is. If you are able to get the right people to help you, it could be quite rewarding in controlling your bipolar condition.

In psychotherapy, you and your doctor would work together to decide the best possible treatment for you. You would be still taking medications during this process. The combination of psychotherapy and medication would be extremely beneficial for your health as well.

When you meet your doctor and talk more about psychotherapy, you would be able to learn more about your bipolar condition. You would be able to find patterns in your condition. As you track and explore the patterns of episodes that you go through, your doctor would better understand what triggers you bipolar condition.

When you start tracking your mood changes, the doctor would be better equip to know what causes your condition in the first place.

One of the best examples is such: If you take medications for another condition that you have, those medications may actually be a reason for your trigger in mood swings and lead to the effect of bipolar.

Other common triggers include emotions. If you have an argument with your loved one, it is only normal to experience a mood swing. However, those who suffer from bipolar would experience a very severe mood swing. Not only do emotional reasons causes such things, physical changes also causes them.

However, identifying these patterns is not enough. Your doctor would also need to find for ways for you to manage these problems. As you learn how to cope with the uncertainties that bipolar brings you. These are all training that you would have to do in order to cope with it.

Always remember that medication alone doesn't bring the help that you'll need to deal with bipolar. You would need to realize that they are dealing with extreme mood swings. Psychotherapy could help you realize that you can cope with whatever that is happening yo you and stop hurting the people that are close to you.

You mustn't ignore the importance of taking your medications. As you realize the extent of what you do during your mood swings and how they are unfounded, you could learn to spot what triggers them and use medication properly.

Please also note that psychotherapy is something which you should do consistently. As you do it more consistently, you allow yourself to be properly coped with bipolar disorder.

# Using Electroconvulsive Therapy

There are certain situations where medications and psychotherapy may not be sufficient to provide them with the relief they need. Another option which would be available for you is electroconvulsive therapy, or more commonly known as ECT.

The people who have to resort to using ECT generally have not responded well to the medication that has been prescribed to them. They may also be serious patients who suffer from severe depression where suicidal thoughts become a constant.

In ECT, the doctor uses electrodes which are placed on your head to start the treatment. He would also give you a muscle relaxer during the treatment. As this is done, you'll be given anesthesia and would feel nothing.

As this is done, the electrodes will admit a tiny amount of electrical current. The current which passes through your brain would cause you to have a seizure. In normal circumstances, the brain seizure is very severe and traumatic but it doesn't happen because you have taken the muscle relaxer. Having taken the muscle relaxer, you would ensure that your body stays still and calm. The current would only pass through your brain for less than a second.

Many people often ask me as to why should this be done. There aren't many answers to that question! During this process of electro-convulsion, your brain reacts in a very different way.

It would change your brain's metabolism significantly as well as the way your blood flows through your brain. It results in a significantly lesser 'feeling' of your depression and makes you feel better. The research that has been done could only prove that it helps depression as well as its symptoms in cases of bipolar disorder. It is still not understood why this happens.

It may be very troublesome to try this therapy. However, you need to remember that the amount of current and the tiny time in which it passes into the brain is very small. Together with the control with muscle relaxers, you end up benefiting from this amazing process, instead of suffering the consequences of it.

# What's Right For You?

There are many types of treatment for bipolar disorder in this book. However, it would be up to you and your doctor to decide which treatment is the best for you. This would be determined from your condition and the severity of it.

It would also take a while to get used to the medications and to obtain the benefits from psychotherapy. During this period, you may even be frustrated by the lack of improvement. Studies have shown the benefits on this combination of medication and psychotherapy to an extent that many patients would see great improvements in their day to day activity.

As you work with your doctor, you would most probably find the same benefit. Always look to work with your doctor as he would have the expertise to help you improve your situation. Stay in constant contact with him about how you are doing.

There is more to it, however.

There is more things that you could do to help improve your condition. We would discuss the other ways you could learn to cope with bipolar.

# Chapter Four: The Reason Why People Struggle With Bipolar Treatment

Some people would not respond well to the combination of medication and psychotherapy. They may stop halfway or simply give up. Some people just don't have the resolve to fight their mind and bodies.

It is simply not the best way for you to follow when you want to care for your condition. However, most bipolar disorder patients would experience this feeling one way or another. This is because antipsychotic medication and mood stabilizers are medication with the most side effects. These side effects can be very difficult for many people to endure. And so, they stop taking it.

It causes a relapse of their symptoms and they end up being hospitalized. They would end up homeless and even be involved with crime. They may even end up being in jail or in hospital. That is why having the right medication is so important.

# When The Patient Doesn't Take The Medication

There are two terms that are used when patients don't take their medication. They are noncompliance and non-adherence. This is not only for those suffering from bipolar but those who suffer from other forms of medical problems as well.

As a matter of fact, many patients that are told to take medications for a long period of time often face a great problem in being consistent with their medications. They would go through a period where they wouldn't want to do it any longer. Many who suffer from asthma, epilepsy or hypertension often feel the same thing of wanting to stop medication.

You need to understand that you wouldn't have to completely stop taking all medications to face a problem. Certain individuals only stop taking some of the medication, not all. However, it has to be noted that partial noncompliance would create just the same problem as cutting off all medications.

There are a few reasons why this happens. They include:

## (1) Lack Of Understanding Of The Illness

The most common reason many patients don't follow through on their medication is simply because they don't understand the illness that they have. Their lack of understanding of bipolar becomes an important issue. When you lack an understanding of the illness, you would tend to not put in enough effort to control it.

In a research done, it has been found that 10 out of 14 patients would stop taking medications because they don't realize the importance of medication in their illness. It has also been found that up to 80 percent of patients only take their medications because their doctors tell them so. They have no idea why they have to.

Therefore, it would be extremely important for you to take time to understand your condition. If you have a loved one with bipolar, you would have to help them by giving them the information you need. Without the essential information, they would not realize the importance of consistently taking their pills each day.

## (2) Dependency On Substances

Dependency on substances is also another major reason why patients don't follow through with their medication.

Many patients put themselves in a terrible position and becoming an incredible health risk due to those substances. Many times, the patient need to make an important choice as to whether to take the medication or continue with their substances like alcohol or drugs.

Of course, it would be extremely unhealthy to consume your medication with other substances as this would cause an unwanted chemical reaction in your body. Mixing alcohol or drugs with medications often could create terrible consequences for your body.

Many patients who have a dependency on drugs or alcohol would find medication very hard. They would instead consume them instead of medications. For this reason, it is advisable for patients to not only use medicinal treatment, but also use substance abuse treatment at the same time.

## (3) Dislike Of The Doctor

This is another common problem that many patients have. It may be because of the attitude of the doctor or simply because the patient finds it hard to communicate with the doctor.

Although this is a common problem, you should never use this as a valid reason for not taking your medication. Not liking your doctor is one thing, not taking your medication is another. You are taking medication because you want to cure yourself. It is for you.

However, if you find it very hard to communicate with your doctor, find for another one. This is as simple as it gets. Nothing like that should ever be a risk towards your health.

## (4) Painful Side Effects

Studies have shown that many people actually stop taking medication because they are afraid of the painful side effects with taking them. However, most people who have this problem are normally those who don't understand their illness well.

Anyone who have understood their illness would know that although medication can be tough, not taking it would be tougher.

The main reason why the medication produces a painful side effect may not because the medication is wrong for you or that your body is weak. It may simply because the dosage that is recommended to you may be wrong. If the dosage is too high or low, it would lead to a number of extreme side effects towards your body.

This is when working with your doctor would pay dividends. Over time, you would be able to get your dosage right so you would be able to improve your overall benefits.

After talking to your doctor about the side effects and all, he would be able to recommend a proper change in dosage. If it seems like its not working, he would later change the medication. It is very common to hear that newer medication are more prone to side effects.

It you talk openly and honestly to your doctor, you could easily find the best medication for your needs as well as the appropriate dosage to control your situation.

# Other Reasons

Many other reasons are used when people stop taking their medication. It has to be clear that medication requires you to have a bit of patience. Many people stop taking medications because they want a quick improvement in their symptoms. It doesn't work that way. Some medication takes a few weeks to see any results at all.

I have even seen people who find it hard to take medications because of their depression. Those that face depression of any kind should have someone to remind them to take their medicine.

Another main issue is the cost of taking medicine. It cannot be denied that many of the recommended medicine isn't cheap. And if you can't afford them, you are better off without it. See if you can get financial aid from the government offices.

There is another reason that may shock you. Some people don't take medicine because they like being that way. They enjoy being in this manic stage. It may be hard to believe but it's true. However, this would only put them at risk in the long term - not only themselves but everyone around them.

# Chapter Five: How To Cope With Bipolar Disorder

Remember that there is no cure for bipolar as yet. All this book is about is how to cope with bipolar disorder. The purpose of this book is to improve your condition.

Don't just expect your condition to improve if you don't put in the effort to deal with it. Reading this book is a good step towards learning more. Don't be a victim towards the circumstances you are dealt with in life. Always take the effort to be strong.

As you realize this, take the time to learn methods to cope with this and learn to have a more positive mentality. Don't expect to make all the changes today. Give yourself some time to work through the changes. The next few pages would be about simple ways which you could learn to improve your quality of life by using these coping techniques. Try them one at a time.

You may be surprised by its simplicity but don't ever write them off. You would never know how powerful the simplest things are.

# Change Your Sleeping Patterns

The way you sleep plays an important role in your bipolar. The amount of sleep you get each night would create chemical changes in your brain that would be beneficial to your condition.

If you desire to improve your condition, always get enough sleep every night. Try to create a sleeping routine and sleep at the same time every night. Creating a sleeping pattern would improve your bipolar symptoms and not put you in a situation of uncertainty.

If you are at a job that require you to sleep at different times in the day, you would need to try to work out a schedule to ensure that regardless of what happens, you still sleep at the same time each day. This is imperative if you are to cope for the long term. It gives your mind the time it needs to be clear and allows you to wake up refreshed.

I have seen patients who have to travel a lot in their jobs and struggle to find a proper sleeping pattern. As such, it would be recommended to ask your doctor for appropriate advice.

# Medications

You should also learn to cope better with the process of taking medication better to make it easier for you. Learn to take your medications even if you feel great. Do whatever your doctor tells you to do when it comes to medication. Even if you have no symptoms, don't stop taking them.

If you feel great after taking medication, don't stop taking them. You need to be consistent with your medication. When you stop consuming them, you simply allow the symptoms to relapse.

You can make the entire process of medication easy by creating a steady schedule which includes the recommended dosage. As an example, once you wake up in the morning, have your breakfast and take your norming pills. If you have to take a second pill for the day, do it after dinner.

Make taking your medication something automated. Something that you do automatically without you thinking at all. When you pair your medication and meals, you will not forget them.

Also purchase a pill organizer if you take more than one pill. This would avoid from you being confused by them. A pill organizer would allow you to portion the right medications and ensure that you wouldn't forget.

One important thing to know is that your medications wouldn't mix well. If you have a cold, consult your doctor about the right cold medications to take with your bipolar medication. You should never mix them with any other substances like alcohol or drugs.

If you meet another doctor and he prescribed a certain medication, ensure that you get the advice from your other doctor. Ask him if it's alright to mix the two medications. Ensure that you discuss with him on the possible consequences of this.

# Stay Active

A crucial thing in managing bipolar disorder is to be organized in your life. If you are someone who is used to working very hard each day, you may need to stop working so hard and cut down on your activity.

Try to control the amount of work you do each day. I'm not talking about being lazy but rather don't overstress yourself in your daily activity. When you start to control the amount you do each day, you will ease the chemical that is in the brain.

Don't be lazy one day and then work your butt off the next. Keeping a consistent energy level helps you control the chemicals in your body.

# Stop Using Drugs Or Alcohol

Many people are very tempted to use alcohol and drugs. Many bipolar patients, when dealing with the symptoms of bipolar, may have this great need to relax. Using drugs and alcohol may be the answer for some people.

The mood swings you feel may be so great that drugs and alcohol is an easy way out. However using these substances with medications can be extremely fatal. And using these substances always brings about more trouble than good.

If you have a great problem with substances, seek help and counseling. It will provide you with the strength you need to overcome that problem. From Alcohol

Anonymous to Twelve Steps, you would find their programs extremely valuable in helping you control the problem.

Using substances should be stopped for good is you want to control your bipolar situation. Even the use of alcohol or caffeine would affect the way your medication reacts to you. Check with your doctor about the right food or medication to use when you are sick.

Remember that anything you take could be a trigger to your mood, even while you are already under medication. They could easily interfere with your sleeping pattern and appetite and put your body in a state which is chemically different.

Most people know that caffeine offers a trigger which keeps them from getting sleepy. If you are someone who needs coffee to keep awake, take decaffeinated coffee instead. However, it is better to completely stop it as just a small dose of coffee may limit the medication effectiveness.

Always be careful about whatever that you take, be it food or medication.

# Get Support

Another important aspect that would determine how you cope would be the support from your family members. As much as you believe you could cope with bipolar with yourself, experience has told me that you can't. In fact I haven't even met someone who is able to cope with their bipolar disorder without proper support from their family members.

This is because you wouldn't realize how your mood swing could easily change from one extreme to another. You would easily lash out at your loved ones with no apparent reason. You may not even realize that.

If you want the support from your family members, the most important step is to be honest with them. The first step is to tell them about your bipolar disorder. As hard as it would seem, your closed ones would be your safety net when things go wrong. They will invariably go wrong, trust me. Having family members who know your condition will allow them to realize certain situation that has gone out of control. A loved one would guide you to get help and will be beside you through ups and downs.

The second step is to understand that you're not the only one in the world with this situation. There are numerous people in the world that are suffering from this situation as well. Because bipolar patients often lash out on their loved ones, their loved ones often feel very stressed when they are with them.

You may not be able to do much about this, but taking the time to inform your loved ones about your situation would go a long way in reducing the stress that they would have in life.

Don't underestimate the help that your loved one could have on your situation. If you don't share with them about your condition, they won't understand why you do certain things. This leads to friction within the family and creates anxious situations. Without educating your family members about your situation, I doubt they could be supportive of your behavior.

Having just knowledge is insufficient. You may also require the family therapist to talk about it. There is a growing trend of family using the services of a family therapist because it helps improve the relationship in the family. It is something which is not only for those people with bipolar, but anyone else who doesn't suffer from this condition. Additionally, family therapy helps turn traumas in family into something which could help bind the family closer.

When a family understands what you are going through, they could strive to improve the condition you are in. They could even help your doctor be informed about your situation and how you react to certain things. They may even assist you in continuing your medication and ensure that you take your medicine consistently.

A supportive family unit is a great tool that would help all bipolar disorder patients. However, it is very common that many people don't use this tool because of embarrassment. If you could go through that phase, you would realize the importance of family in assisting you through this condition.

# Look To Reduce Stress

Many people know that stress creates a lot of problems in their lives. However, a big number of people believe that it seems impossible to reduce stress.

It is very important to look at your life and see during which periods that you are stressed. Look to identify those periods when stress leads to mood swings or even extreme behavior that puts you in risk of lashing out and being out of control.

If you see yourself as someone who is constantly pushing yourself to achieve more in your career, you would most probably create numerous symptoms of bipolar. You would become more stressed and out of control. If that happen, you would put yourself in a position where you can't work optimally or even putting your career at risk. You would not be able to benefit from your hard work and would have fewer opportunities.

You could instead work on a steady schedule and don't over-stress yourself. If you are better able in dealing with stress, it is without a doubt that you would accomplish more.

These are some tips that would help you reduce stress at work:

- **Get Enough Rest.** Always look to sleep at the same time every day. From there, you would be able to monitor your sleeping patterns, thus reducing mood swings.
- **Work The Same Hours Daily.** When you work a predictable and

steady schedule, you would be able to lessen mood swings in your life.

- **Always Take Time Off.** When you take quality time off to improve your health, you would be able to perform better and reduce the stress that you have.

- **If You Suffer From Mood Swings, Stop.** This is subjective but you should talk to your doctor if you should stop working if you suffer mood swings. However, it cannot be doubted that this would be a great thing to do if you suffer from mood swings.

- **Don't Work In Environment That Are Too Stressed.** This may be a situation that you feel is hard for you to control, but this is perhaps the most important decision to make. If you feel your job is too stressful, look to find another job. You would never know how bipolar may be triggered by certain situations.

- **Deal With Small Problems Straight Away.** Many problems start off small and becoming bigger with time. Small problems turn into big ones if not dealt with immediately. If you make it a habit to handle problems quickly, you can reduce the stress that would be on you ultimately.

Reducing stress is perhaps the best thing to do if you want to control your bipolar disorder. This reduces mood swings from stress. Learning to spot stressful situation would assist you with that. It would eventually pay off.

# Be On The Lookout For Signs

The best tool to help you in coping with your bipolar condition is to learn to watch for the subtle signs of the mood swings onset. This early warning signs could be seen before it become full blown swings.

As you pay attention to this, you could have a number of benefits that would come from observing and taking action on them. Your doctor only has a mere idea about what would happen during your mood swings. You have to remember that each person is unique and it provides a challenge to your doctor to decide for you. Different people move from depressive to manic symptoms differently and in different situations.

If you are able to notice your mood changing faster, you could take action to deal with it faster. As you do it faster, the faster you can help yourself.

There are several warning signs. These are things that could be small but ultimately be the predictor of a larger mood swing. Learn to notice these changes immediately.

- **Energy Levels Depleting.** A strong indicator is your fluctuations in your energy levels. Most of the time, mania is a situation where you have excessive energy, while depressive is when you have lower energy levels.
- **Changes In Sleeping Patterns.** You should always be on a regular sleeping pattern. If you realize that you aren't sleeping as regularly as you should, it is a predictor of your mood swings.

- **Losing Interest In Sex.** Many bipolar patients would encounter times where they wouldn't want any sort of sexual intercourse. It may seem normal but patients of bipolar would have an increased change from wanting and not wanting sex.
- **Lowered Self-Esteem**. This is something that you wouldn't be able to judge well. It would depend on your loved ones to determine when that happens. When it seems like your self-esteem gets lower, it could be a sign that you are heading for a depressive symptom arising.
- **Losing Concentration.** Losing concentration is a sign that you are having lower energy levels. If you struggle to work and get your work

done, it may be a sign that your depressive symptoms may be coming.

- **Changes In Your Exterior Outlook.** In many bipolar patients that I have seen, I see a pattern where they feel the need to change how they look. You may suddenly dislike the way you look or suddenly want a change. This is a major sign of mood swings because emotions are often correlated with the way you dress.

- **Changes In Your Thinking.** If you are thinking about certain things for too long a period, it may be a major sign that you are having a mood swing. For example, if you are constantly thinking about suicide, you need to seek help instantly.

These early signs of your mood swing can be great tools to assist you in spotting the mood changes. However, one of the biggest problems with this is that many people wouldn't even be spot this fast enough on their own. They may see that these changes as their everyday lifestyle.

It is because of this that family should help the patient spot the signs and assist you in getting through them. When you spot the changes (as mentioned by your family), you could look to make changes immediately.

If you experience this mood changes, contact your doctor quickly to obtain the relief you need. They can not only play a role in assisting you physically, but also offer supportive advice that you need and helping you spot mood swings.

# Keep In Constant Contact With Your Doctor

There are people that I have met who disliked going to the doctor because they seem so negative and always have bad things to say, but it is extremely important to keep them informed. If you tell them what is going on and how you feel, he would be able to decide better on your condition.

When you face these situations, you would have to immediately meet your doctor:

- When your family notices mood swings in you.
- When you feel that you would have a mood swing soon.
- When you feel that you are having a mood swing.
- When you feel suicidal or feel despair.

- When you feel that your medications are not working.

The doctor would assist you in learning how to cope with these situations. They may also make medicinal changes that could act as a way to improve your well-being. When you keep your doctor informed about your situation, you are better able to monitor your symptoms. He would learn the patterns and notice the things that trigger your emotional reactions.

This would lead to greater benefits for you. This would include helping you avoid certain situations that would lead to lesser mood swings in your life. Learning to cope with bipolar is a must for a patient. If you take a look at your life now, you will see that things could be changed. You would immediately improve your well-being.

*Are you sleeping and eating well?*

*Are you aware of your early warning signs?*

These are excellent questions in improving your overall well-being. As you learn to cope better with bipolar, you would instantly feel better.

In the next chapters, you would learn a few other ways to cope with them, including using support groups. This would be discussed thoroughly in the next chapter.

# Chapter Six: How Support Groups Can Help You

Many people have this negative perception about support groups. They hate them and feel that people who attend such support groups as weak and useless. You need to understand why you have this misconception. Why is it hard for you to attend a support group? Or do you hate admitting that something in your life is wrong?

It may be because you are unused to the fact with admitting that you are weak and needs help. However, you should note that if you surround yourself with people who struggle with the same challenges like you do, you would instantly feel better.

Support groups assist you and they help improve the quality of life of the people around you to understand what you are facing. Coping with bipolar disorder is not easy and it extremely challenging. You will need to learn how to do it. You could learn to do this with the help of others who face the same situations like you do.

Support groups are incredible in a sense that you would be with people that offer a certain care that family and friends wouldn't be able to give you. Not even your doctor would be able to help you with that. Being with other people who struggle with the same thing not only help you cope but would also inspire you to be better. They give you more hope and understanding.

# Do You Have A Support Group?

Support groups are more than just those people who have the same issues that you have. It also includes your family and friends. Whoever is in your circle of support depends on you. You would need to strive to provide yourself with an environment that you could improve your bipolar situation.

Now, you may have a family to support your needs. You may also have a group of medical practitioners that assist you with medical assistance.

However, that isn't sufficient. Friends should also be part of that group. It may be very uncomfortable for you to provide personal information about themselves, but if you are open enough to them, it will do you a great deal of help.

Having a true friend who stays by you and assist you in coping with your situation may be all that you need when you face a tough situation. Think about telling your loved ones about what is happening to you. It would only help you in the long run.

What's more, if they have experienced the same thing, they could give you advice about how to handle certain situations. You could also give them advice, thus making you a better friend as well.

# Getting External Support

Having a family around you would undoubtedly help you a lot with coping with bipolar. However, you mustn't ignore the power of having outside support.

There are professional groups that could be found in hospitals or psychiatric facilities that you could meet up to discuss about bipolar. Ask your doctor for suggestions. He would be able to locate one which suits you needs, based on the right age group and locality.

The support groups give you professional attention. You would be able to share the ups and downs of your life with others. They provide great emotional support and may also be a great source of knowledge on knowing how to cope with different situations that you may face in your day to day tasks.

You can't expect to isolate yourself if you have bipolar disorder. Therapy groups would provide you with the emotional support that would seem crucial for your improvement. It helps to know a group of people who face the same things as you are. You will not feel alone in what you are facing.

The very fact that you could attend a group like this should be a great factor in improving your condition. The environment which allows you to talk about your problem reduces the amount of time between your mood swings. Talking about your problems would prove to be an excellent way to release the stresses associated with them.

You would not only be able to help yourself but you would also be able to help other patients with the same problems. No one would be able to understand how difficult it is except for the people who have experienced those feelings themselves.

As you utilize support from your family, friends, professionals and outside support; you could gain a great level of understanding and emotional support. Bipolar may be tough for you, but knowing that you have a group of people being with you would go a long way towards fighting it.

If you want to get a book that allows your spouse better cope with it, check out this link:

http://bipolar-spouse.wellbeingvalley.com

# Chapter Seven: Monitoring Symptoms Using A Mood Chart

There are many ways that you can cope with bipolar. However nothing is more important than monitoring your symptoms. We have discusses why you need to look out for the early signs of bipolar, but it is also imperative that you see changes in your treatment.

If you are to monitor your own bipolar treatment, you should be using a mood chart. A mood chart is able to track the way you feel on a given day. As you keep track of this, you would be able to see the ups and downs of your condition.

A professional doctor may ask you to keep a mood chart. This is especially so at the start of your treatment. However, you may want to continue with it for a longer period because it helps you and the people who are close to you in spotting your mood changes.

A mood chart is something like a simple diary that you could use to keep track of your changes in your moods, feelings, things you do and how you sleep. It would be an incredibly effective tool if you sue it well.

For starters, you should ensure that you jot these down:

1) **How You Feel That Day**. See if you have any significantly feeling changes. Record anything that makes you in a good or bad mood.

2) **Any Activities That You Do**. IF you have to work, jot it down. If you are spending time with friends or relatives, jot it down as well. Writing down the things you do go a long way in spotting the triggers to spot mood swings.
3) **Any Life Changes/Events** That Are Significance.
4) **Sleep Patterns**. This is very important for bipolar patients because sleep is a big trigger in your emotions.
5) **Medication As Well As Its Side Effects**. Notice the feelings that you would have when you take those medications.

Although you may seem like you have normal day, you must write it down. This helps to create a writing habit and determine any changes that you have made in your daily life. You wouldn't incorporate a lot of details on most days. However, if you find yourself in a situation where there is something which triggers you, you need to write in more detail.

In the market, there are quite a number of charts that could be extremely useful for you. Talk to your doctor about the right one which would help you the most. This would provide you with the convenience of writing as well as detecting your triggers.

You can even have a virtual diary which you keep on your computer. This is very flexible. However, the key is to be consistent. The rewards from this are unimaginable.

# Final Notes On Bipolar

Bipolar disorder is something which would affect you your entire life. It is something which affects millions of people around the world. However, most of them go on and live a normal life if they learn the right coping skills to empower themselves.

Always remember that you have a choice. You could choose to live a happy and fulfilling life or you can continue to suffer from it. But remember, you are not the only one suffering. Your loved ones suffer as well. They may even suffer more than you do.

The road to a better life can be filled with potholes – situations where you need to suffer and lead to giving certain things up but the reward is that you live a more fulfilling life.

All these coping techniques are just the start of your journey. You need to consistently practice them if you want to improve your life. Reading this book isn't sufficient without practice.

You are a worthy person. Put in the effort to change. Your fulfilling life starts today and it starts with you.

# Resources

To get more information on Bipolar Disorder, check out these links. These information would be great if you would like to better cope with bipolar.

1) http://bipolar-spouse.wellbeingvalley.com
Do you have a bipolar husband or wife?
Dealing with a bipolar spouse isn't easy and this guide provides the guide about how to help your partner and to better cope with it yourself.

2) http://bipolar.wellbeingvalley.com
If you want to know more about bipolar, this guide is great for you. If you want to know more about bipolar, this is about the best book you could have.

Made in the USA
Columbia, SC
11 October 2023